A Woman's Guide to Optimum Health

by **Sherry Torkos**, B.Sc.Phm., Pharmacist

John Wiley & Sons Canada, Ltd.

Live Well: A Woman's Guide to Optimum Health
ISBN-13: 978-0-470-84078-8
ISBN-10: 0-470-84078-1

Production Credits
Cover design: Barefoot Creative Inc.
Interior text design: Adrian So
Cover photography: Bryn Gladding Photography
Wiley Bicentennial Logo: Richard J. Pacifico
Printer: Tri-Graphic Printing Ltd.

John Wiley & Sons Canada, Ltd.
6045 Freemont Blvd.
Mississauga, Ontario
L5R 4J3

Printed in Canada
2 3 4 5 TRI 10 09 08 07

Table of Contents

Introduction

As women we tend to define ourselves by our roles in life. We are mothers, we are wives, we are daughters, we are employees, and we are our own person last. In the busyness of life, we forget that we are important too. It's natural for us to nurture others. We can be counted on to lend a helping hand to a friend, make a healthy meal for an ailing mother, stand in a cold arena to cheer on our little hockey player, or book that annual doctor's visit for our husband.

When we become overly absorbed in caring for others, we tend to disregard or "put off" the time and care we need. We can fool ourselves into believing that our time will come when our children move out, we retire, and our parents pass on, but waiting has consequences. Continuing to sacrifice for the sake of others can leave us facing serious health issues and struggling to manage emotionally and perhaps even financially.

The Time is NOW
Your health is like a retirement fund. The sooner you implement the program and begin making deposits, the quicker the benefits begin to build. And so, it also stands to reason that the more substantial the contributions, the more substantial or "healthier" the result.

What are the fundamental principles for optimal health? Quite simply: eat well, exercise regularly, and take time to relax and to have fun. We have heard this formula before. However, in today's fast-paced world, weaving these elements into a solid and sustained LIFESTYLE is vital to your enjoyment of life.

In the pages to come we will discuss nutrition, exercise, stress management, and the importance of sleep. We will then take a look at five important areas of concern for women in Canada: heart health, breast health, osteoporosis, menopause, and weight management. We will examine risk factors, symptoms, management or treatment of the condition, and, most importantly, how to prevent or minimize the effects of each. Lastly, we will discuss the importance of ensuring a healthy financial future.

Part One

NUTRITION FOR OPTIMUM HEALTH

The food choices we make on a daily basis have an impact on both our physical and emotional health. In this chapter you will find 10 dietary principles for optimal health, energy, and well-being.

Make Quality Food Choices

Fresh, natural, unprocessed foods should form the basis of your diet.

- Carbohydrates such as whole grains (brown rice, multi-grain breads), legumes, vegetables, and fruits provide essential vitamins, minerals, fibre, and a readily available source of energy. Avoid refined flour products (white bread, pasta, rice) as these foods have lower nutritional value and minimal fibre.
- Protein is essential to help build and maintain muscle. It provides energy and is used by the body to make hormones and enzymes. Good dietary sources include free-range and organic meat and poultry, legumes, nuts, seeds, and tofu.
- Fat is necessary for the growth and development of many organs, in particular the brain. It provides energy, aids vitamin absorption, and is used to make hormones. Health-promoting fats are found in fish, nuts, seeds, and plant oils (hemp, flaxseed, canola, olive, sunflower, and safflower). Avoid saturated fats and trans fats as they are linked to heart disease.

Enjoy Variety

To get a broad range of nutrients in your diet, enjoy a variety of foods rather than sticking to your favourites. This is particularly important with vegetables and fruits as their nutrient profiles vary greatly. Experiment with new foods and recipes, and try to reintroduce previously disliked foods.

Practice Moderation

To prevent overeating, control your portion sizes and eat slowly. Canada's Food Guide to Healthy Eating recommends adults consume five to 12 servings of grains, five to 10 servings of vegetables and fruits, two to four servings of milk products, and two to three servings of meat and alternatives. A serving equals one piece of fruit, one cup of raw or ½ cup cooked vegetables, one slice of bread, ½ cup of cooked rice or pasta, or 50 to 100 grams of meat.

Eating slowly allows time for your stomach to send a message to your brain that you are full. Chew your food thoroughly to allow for proper digestion. It should take you 20 to 30 minutes to eat a meal.

Eat Small, Frequent Meals

Try to eat three small meals and two snacks daily. This will improve metabolism (calorie burning) and blood sugar balance, which improves energy and mood.

Don't skip meals, even if trying to lose weight, since this causes fatigue, poor concentration, sluggish metabolism, and triggers food cravings. Breakfast is especially important to give you energy in the morning. If you aren't very hungry, have a light meal such as yogurt and berries or a protein shake.

Drink Plenty of Water

Water helps regulate body temperature, remove wastes, and transport nutrients through the body. To keep your body well hydrated, drink two to three litres of pure water daily. Intense physical activity and heat exposure increase water loss and therefore increase the need for more fluids.

Boost Fibre Intake

Most Canadians are getting only a fraction of the recommended 25 to 38 grams of fibre per day. Fibre reduces your risk of diabetes, heart disease, and certain cancers. Plus, it keeps your bowels regular, improves blood sugar control, and plays a role in weight management. Dietary fibre is found in fruits, vegetables, beans, seeds, and whole grains such as wheat and oat bran. If your diet is lacking in fibre, consider a supplement.

Cut Down on Salt; Boost Potassium

Salt (sodium) helps maintain fluid balance and aids muscle and nerve function. However, excess amounts can contribute to high blood pressure, especially in older individuals, those of black-African descent, and those with diabetes and kidney disease.

The Institute of Medicine recommends adults consume 3.8 grams of salt daily to replace the amount lost through sweat. The maximum recommended amount is 5.8 grams daily; most adults regularly consume more than this amount.

Salt is naturally present in dairy, seafood, vegetables, and grains. However, most of our salt comes from processed foods such as deli meats, condiments (ketchup), sauces (soy), snack foods (chips, pretzels), and the salt shaker. Cut back on these foods and season food with herbs or flavoured oils and vinegars instead.

Potassium also plays a role in regulating fluid balance, nerve and muscle function, and blood pressure. Most Canadians consume less than the recommended amount of potassium, which is 4.7 grams daily. To boost potassium intake, eat more bananas, oranges and orange juice, avocados, peaches, and tomatoes.

Minimize Sugar

Excessive sugar intake is linked to diabetes, obesity, elevated triglycerides, tooth decay, poor immune function, and other health problems. The World Health Organization recommends restricting consumption of added sugar—including sugar from honey, syrups and fruit juices—to below 10 percent of daily calories.

To satisfy a craving for sweets, have fruit (fresh or dried). Fruit contains natural sugar (fructose) but it also provides vitamins, minerals, and fibre. Mashed bananas or apple sauce are great substitutions for sugar in baked goods. Stevia, a natural sweetener obtained from a plant, is another good substitute for sugar. It can provide up to 300 times the sweetening power of sugar without the calories.

Cut Down on Caffeine

A high intake of caffeine (more than three cups per day) can promote calcium loss from bones, increase blood pressure, and cause insomnia, irritability, and anxiety. Drip coffee has the highest caffeine content. Try switching your coffee or cola to herbal tea, or limit intake to no more than two cups daily.

Limit Alcohol

Heavy and chronic drinking (more than three drinks per day) is linked to liver and cardiovascular disease, pancreatitis, immune system depression, increased risk of cancer, brain damage, sexual dysfunction, infertility, and malnutrition.

Moderate alcohol consumption is a different story. Research has found that one to two drinks daily reduces the risk of heart disease, likely due to its ability to increase HDL (good) cholesterol and reduce blood clotting. Some alcohol also contains antioxidants, as seen with red wine and dark beer. The bottom line—limit your intake to one to two drinks per day.

EXERCISE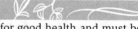

Regular exercise and physical activity is essential for good health and must be part of your daily life. Numerous studies have shown that regular exercise cuts your risk of chronic, debilitating diseases such as heart disease (by reducing cholesterol and blood pressure), osteoporosis (by strengthening bones), cancer (by supporting immune function), and diabetes (by improving blood sugar control). Exercise is essential for developing and maintaining a healthy body weight, flexibility, and muscular strength. Plus, it offers emotional benefits. Exercise reduces stress and anxiety and improves sleep and overall emotional well-being.

Regardless of your health status, age, or current fitness level, there are activities that you can do to improve your health.

Cardiovascular (Aerobic) Exercise

Cardiovascular activities are those that involve large muscle groups and increase our heart rate, such as brisk walking, swimming, biking, aerobics, and dancing. These activities burn calories and improve heart and lung function.

If you are currently not exercising, then start slowly. Try exercising for five minutes on your first day, and increase gradually. Aim for 30 minutes to an hour, five times per week.

Resistance Exercise

Activities that use resistance to challenge your muscles increase strength, endurance, and muscle mass. They also strengthen bones. Examples include weightlifting, using exercise machines or bands/tubes, or using your own body weight to do exercises such as lunges, squats, and push-ups. These activities are particularly important for older adults because they help prevent the muscle and bone loss that occurs with aging.

Aim for 20 to 30 minutes of resistance activities three to four times per week. Vary your activities and routine to continually challenge your muscles.

Stretching

Stretching helps to improve flexibility and joint health and to prevent soreness after a workout. Spend about five to 10 minutes stretching all of your muscles. Stretch slowly and gently, breathe deeply, and hold each position for at least 10 seconds.

How Much Exercise Do I Need?

The Institute of Medicine recommends that adults and children spend a total of at least one hour daily in moderately intense physical activity. There are plenty of ways to build more activity into your daily life, whether it is short walks in the morning, using the stairs instead of the elevator, or doing housework with vigour. Every little bit helps.

Creating Your Fitness Program

If you have been sedentary all your life, the prospect of getting active may be intimidating, so take it slowly.

- Consult with your doctor before you start an exercise program, especially if you have any health conditions or are taking medication.
- Set reasonable goals and be consistent with your exercise program.
- Don't expect overnight results. Gradually increase the duration and intensity of your workout; you will see (and feel) the benefits.
- Be sure to drink lots of water during and after your workout.
- Make time to stretch your muscles after you workout.
- For guidance on proper exercise technique and help in designing a workout, see a certified personal trainer.

• Keep your motivation high: get a workout partner, vary your activities, and have fun.

SLEEP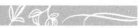

Sleep is one of the body's most basic needs for health and well-being, yet nearly half of all adults report having difficulty sleeping.

While we think of sleep as a relaxing and passive state, there is actually a lot happening in our body during sleep. This is a time when our major organs and regulatory systems repair and regenerate, and important hormones are released.

An occasional sleepless night is not a concern, but persistent difficulty falling asleep, waking during the night, or waking feeling tired could indicate insomnia—a condition that can affect both our physical and emotional well-being.

How Much Sleep Do We Need?

The exact amount of sleep needed varies among individuals, but is thought to be between seven and nine hours. Lack of sleep, particularly deep sleep, not only makes us feel tired, but also causes memory loss, poor concentration, depression, headache, irritability, increased response to stress, high blood pressure, depressed immune function, and low libido.

Causes of Poor Sleep

There are many factors that can affect the quality of sleep—stress, medical problems (depression, anxiety), medications, alcohol, poor nutrition, noise, light, the need to go to the bathroom during the night, and poor sleep hygiene (going to bed at different times). If you have persistent difficulty sleeping, it is important to consult with your doctor.

Tips for a Better Night's Rest

• Establish a regular sleeping routine.
• Do relaxing activities before bed. Read a book, have a warm bath, or meditate.
• Reserve your bedroom for intimacy and sleep. Don't watch TV, read, or do computer work in your bedroom.
• Make your bedroom dark, quiet, and comfortable.
• Avoid caffeine (coffee, tea, pop, chocolate) and smoking within six hours of bedtime.
• Avoid alcohol before bed. It may help you fall asleep, but drinking alcohol causes nighttime waking and reduces sleep quality.
• Exercise regularly, early in the day.
• If you work shifts or travel to different time zones, try a supplement of melatonin (a hormone naturally secreted in response to darkness).

Our bodies do not maintain a sleep reserve. Depriving yourself of adequate sleep on a regular basis can take a toll on your health. Considering the vital role that sleep plays in our well-being, devoting seven to nine hours per night should be a priority.

STRESS MANAGEMENT

Stress has become a common complaint of modern living. We take on too much, worry about health and wealth, and feel overwhelmed and "stressed-out" on a regular basis. Nearly half of all adults suffer the adverse health effects of stress such as muscle tension, anxiety, and high blood pressure.

Understanding Stress

Stress as defined by Hans Selye, a Canadian physician who studied the effects of stress and anxiety, is "the non-specific response of the body to any demand placed upon it." He claimed that it isn't stress that harms us but *distress*—a phenomenon that occurs when we have prolonged emotional stress and don't deal with it in a positive manner. In other words, stress is not an external force but rather how we react internally to a trigger such as traffic, deadlines at work, children fighting, or any event that we perceive as stressful.

Stress and Disease

In response to stress, the body releases stress hormones—adrenaline, noradrenaline, and cortisol—to prepare the body to fight. Heart rate, blood pressure, and lung tone increase. This innate reaction served us well centuries ago when we had to fight off wild animals and protect our villages. Stress today is very different. It is chronic rather than occasional, and stems primarily from psychological rather than physical threats.

Stress has far-reaching effects on our health. It is linked to heart disease, cancer, diabetes, high cholesterol and blood pressure, anxiety, depression, memory loss, insomnia, muscle tension, obesity, fatigue, sexual dysfunction, and many other problems.

Managing Your Stress

It is absolutely crucial to find ways to cope with stress effectively. Identify your stressors and then explore ways of changing your responses to those situations. Rethink your natural reaction, avoid known stressful situations, and utilize the following stress-reducing strategies.

Meditation

Meditation is the practice of focusing the mind and consciously relaxing the body for a sustained period. Sit in a quiet, comfortable area and close your eyes. Starting with your feet and working your way up, relax all of your muscles. Clear your mind and focus your attention on your breathing or on a calming image or sound. Breathe in slowly and deeply and then out. Do this for ten or twenty minutes. You can do this when feeling stressed, or make a habit of meditating once or twice a day for better health and relaxation.

Breathing Techniques

Taking slow controlled breaths is a great way to promote calming. Place the tip of your tongue against the roof of your mouth just behind your front teeth. Begin by exhaling through your mouth around your tongue, then close your mouth and inhale deeply through your nose for four seconds. Hold your breath for five seconds, and then completely exhale out through your mouth, making a whoosh sound. Repeat this cycle four or five times. This technique can be done any time and anywhere.

Exercise

Regular exercise helps reduce stress, promote calming, and improve both physical and emotional well-being. It also increases blood flow to muscles. Walking, cycling, yoga, and Tai Chi are just a few activities to consider.

Visualization

This technique involves concentrating your mind on images that make you feel calm and relaxed. Close your eyes, take a few deep breaths, and visualize a picture or event that makes you feel calm and centered. Focus on the details: for example, focus on the sounds, images, and scents.

Other Considerations

- Massage and acupuncture promote relaxation of the body and mind.
- Supplements that help with stress include theanine, B vitamins, and magnesium.
- Taking on too much leads to feeling overwhelmed and pressed for time. Make time to do nothing but relax.
- Negative people, places, and events can create unnecessary stress.
- Sharing your feelings and concerns with friends, family, or a therapist can help you to feel supported.

Dealing more effectively with stress will bring many health rewards, including fewer physical and emotional ailments and an overall improved well-being. Identify the areas where you are struggling, seek help, and work on adopting positive changes.

Part Two

WOMEN AND HEART HEALTH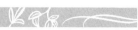

Heart disease, also known as cardiovascular disease, refers to diseases of the blood vessels and heart. Heart disease is the leading cause of death among Canadian women. However, there are many ways to keep your heart healthy and to reduce your risk of heart disease.

Heart Disease

The most common types of heart disease are:

Coronary Artery Disease (CAD)

Also known as atherosclerosis or hardening of the arteries, CAD occurs when the coronary arteries become narrow, thick, and hard due to a buildup of plaque. The supply of oxygen-rich blood to the heart is reduced, leading to chest pain (angina). If the coronary arteries become completely blocked and the flow of blood is cut off, a heart attack (myocardial infarction) occurs and this results in damage to the heart muscle.

Hypertension

Hypertension is also known as high blood pressure. Blood pressure is a measure of the force exerted by your blood against the artery walls. Normal blood pressure is below 120/80. The top (systolic) number represents the pressure when your heart contracts and pushes blood through the arteries. The bottom (diastolic) number is the lowest pressure when the heart relaxes between beats. Blood pressure that is consistently greater than 140/90 is considered high.

High blood pressure can damage the artery walls causing scarring and plaque buildup (atherosclerosis), and it also strains the heart and kidneys. Untreated high blood pressure places you at high risk for a heart attack or stroke. *According to the Heart and Stroke Foundation, 18 percent of Canadian women have high blood pressure, yet up to half aren't aware they have a problem.*

Stroke

Stroke refers to a sudden loss of brain function. There are two forms: ischemic stroke occurs when there is an interruption of flow of blood to the brain; hemorrhagic stroke occurs when blood vessels rupture in the brain. Both forms cause brain cells in the affected area to die, resulting in impairment of speech, movement, memory, thinking, and the ability to read and write. The longer the brain goes without oxygen and nutrients, the greater the risk of permanent damage.

Congestive Heart Failure

Congestive heart failure is defined by a weakening of the pumping action of the heart, which reduces the delivery of blood and oxygen to the body. This can result in a backup of fluid in your lungs, legs, or other parts of your body.

How Is Heart Disease Different in Women?

Years ago it was thought that heart disease was the same for women and men. Today we know that there are unique factors in women:

- Symptoms of a heart attack can be different for women. They may include fatigue, nausea, or pain in the shoulder, neck, or stomach, rather than the typical chest pain and shortness of breath.
- Heart disease more often affects women later in life than men. Nonetheless, younger women who have heart disease often do less well than men because it can be unrecognized by both the woman and her doctor.
- Women often delay going to the doctor, or fail to seek treatment altogether.
- Women are often treated less aggressively than men, and women's symptoms may be dismissed as related to anxiety or emotions.
- Women are more likely than men to die after a first heart attack.
- Standard testing (angiogram) may not pick up heart disease in women due to differences in the formation of plaque. In women, plaque may form more smoothly against the artery walls, whereas in men it clumps up and is more apparent with testing. In addition, in some women the plaque buildup may be in the small vessels of the coronary arteries, which cannot be seen by the angiogram.
- Women have been under-represented in the studies used to set the standards for detection and treatment of heart disease.
- Women are more affected by stress, which is one of the common risk factors for heart disease. Stress causes the arteries to go into spasm and can trigger a heart attack. Women today have increased responsibilities—managing careers and taking care of the family and the home—and often put the needs of others ahead of their needs.

Risk Factors We Can Control

- Smoking: Women who smoke have two to three times the risk of heart disease; exposure to second hand smoke is also a risk factor.
- Inactivity: Not getting enough physical activity (couch potato lifestyle) doubles your risk.
- Stress: Increases in blood pressure, cholesterol, and the formation of clots are all associated with both stress and heart disease.

- Carrying excess weight: Being overweight increases blood pressure, cholesterol, and the risk of diabetes—all factors that also increase your risk of heart disease.
- Poor dietary choices: Studies indicate that a high intake of saturated and trans fats or a low intake of fibre can increase the risk of heart disease.
- Excess alcohol consumption: Drinking too much alcohol (especially binge drinking) raises blood pressure and increases the risk of heart disease. On the other hand, some research has found that a moderate intake (one drink per day) can reduce the risk.
- High blood pressure: High blood pressure significantly increases the risk of heart disease.
- High cholesterol: High cholesterol doubles a woman's risk of heart disease.
- Diabetes: Diabetes is an even bigger risk for heart disease in women than in men.

Studies have shown that you can reduce the risk of heart disease by following a heart-healthy lifestyle. That includes eating well, being physically active, maintaining a healthy weight, and reducing stress.

Risk Factors Beyond Our Control
- Age: Advanced age increases risk. For women, the risk of heart disease increases rapidly after age 55.
- Family history: Having a parent or grandparent with heart disease early in life (before age 65) could indicate a genetic predisposition.
- Ethnic background: Those of South Asian, Aboriginal/First Nations, Inuit, or black-African descent are at increased risk for some types of heart disease.

Emerging Risk Factors
In recent years, research has identified other factors that may increase your risk of heart disease:
- Homocysteine: Homocysteine is an amino acid made by the body during normal metabolism. Studies suggest that elevated homocysteine increases the risk of heart disease by causing damage to the lining of the arteries and promoting clots. Homocysteine metabolism is controlled by vitamins B6, B12, and folic acid. A deficiency of these nutrients can increase levels; likewise, supplementing with these nutrients can lower homocysteine levels.
- C-Reactive Protein (CRP): CRP is a marker of inflammation, which is a factor in the development of atherosclerosis. High CRP levels are correlated with an increased risk of heart attack and stroke. If you are at risk of heart disease your doctor may check your CRP levels.

An Aspirin a Day?
While aspirin is widely recommended for primary prevention of heart disease in men, recent studies have shown that for women there are more risks than benefits associated with its use. It is still recommended for secondary prevention (for those who are diagnosed with heart disease) and for prevention of ischemic stroke in women over 65 who are at high risk.

The Power of Prevention

If you have heart disease or are at risk, consider all of the healthy lifestyle choices outlined in the Part One of this book, as well as the following specific recommendations:

- Have your blood pressure and cholesterol regularly checked, and discuss your results with your doctor.
- Eat a heart-healthy diet that includes colourful fruits and vegetables, soy foods, whole grains, healthy fats (fish), and adequate protein.
- Swap green tea for coffee (green tea contains antioxidants that offer benefits for the heart).
- Get regular exercise and maintain a healthy body weight.
- Manage your stress levels with regular exercise, breathing techniques, and meditation.
- Don't smoke, and avoid second-hand smoke. If you are currently a smoker, talk to your pharmacist about smoking cessation aids. There are many products and programs available today to help you kick the habit.

Supplements

There are many nutritional supplements that have been studied for their heart-health benefits. Here are some options to consider:

- Antioxidants: Numerous studies have shown that those who consume antioxidant-rich diets have lower rates of heart disease. It is thought that antioxidants may function best when taken together, as they offer synergistic and protective effects in combination. Consider taking a product that contains natural vitamin E, vitamin C, beta-carotene, and selenium.
- Coenzyme Q10 is another antioxidant that has been widely studied and found to offer specific benefits for helping to lower blood pressure and cholesterol.
- Vitamins B6, B12, and folic acid lower homocysteine levels. Vitamin B3 (niacin) is sometimes prescribed to lower cholesterol levels.
- Soluble fibre such as oat bran helps lower cholesterol.
- Omega-3 fatty acids in fish oil can help lower blood pressure, reduce atherosclerosis, and protect against heart attack.

• Garlic helps lower blood pressure and cholesterol, reduces clotting, and prevents plaque formation in the arteries. Most research has been conducted on aged garlic extract.

Consult with your pharmacist for help in choosing supplements. Keep in mind that supplements are not intended to replace prescription medication. In most cases they can be taken along with your prescribed therapies, but it is always wise to check with your pharmacist to avoid any interactions.

Taking It to Heart

While heart disease is the greatest health threat that women face, there is much that we can do to prevent it. The majority of the risk factors are under our control, so we can take the necessary steps—eating healthily, exercising regularly, not smoking, and reducing stress—to cut our risk of heart disease and improve our health.

BREAST HEALTH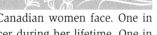

Breast cancer is the most feared disease that Canadian women face. One in nine women is expected to develop breast cancer during her lifetime. One in 27 will die of it. In 2006, an estimated 22,200 women will be diagnosed with breast cancer, and 5,300 will die of it.

While these figures are startling, the good news is that since 1993 the incidence of breast cancer has stabilized and death rates have declined steadily. With early detection, improved treatments, and knowledge of prevention, women today are doing much better in the battle against breast cancer.

Risk Factors

There are a number of factors that have been found to increase the risk of developing breast cancer:

• Age: Risk increases with age.
• Family history: Having a mother, sister, or daughter diagnosed with breast cancer before menopause, or a family history of uterine, colorectal, or ovarian cancer increases your risk.
• Previous breast disorders: Risk increases if you have had previous biopsies showing abnormal cells.
• Hormone replacement therapy: Taking HRT for more than five years increases your risk.
• Excess weight: Even a small amount of excess weight (five kg or 11 lbs) is associated with increased risk, especially among postmenopausal women.
• No pregnancies: Not becoming pregnant or having a first pregnancy after age 30 increases risk.

- Early menstruation: Beginning to menstruate before age 12 increases risk.
- Late menopause: Beginning menopause at age 55 or older increases risk.
- Radiation (X-rays): Exposure of the breasts to high levels of radiation increases risk.
- Dense breast tissue: Dense breast tissue increases risk.

There is also some evidence linking alcohol intake, oral contraceptives, smoking, and a lack of physical activity to breast cancer. Breast implants have not been found to increase the risk for breast cancer.

It is important to note that most women with breast cancer do not have a family history of the disease or any of the identified risks. There remain many unanswered questions surrounding the underlying causes of breast cancer.

Signs and Symptoms

While detecting a lump in the breast is the most common sign of breast cancer, other signs might include: a lump or swelling in the armpit; dimpling, puckering, or thickening of the skin on the breast; inverted nipples; changes in breast size or shape; redness, swelling, and increased warmth in the breast; and crusting or scaling of the nipple.

Not all lumps are breast cancer. In fact, most that are found are not cancer. A condition called *Fibrocystic Breast Disease* causes lumps in the breast. These lumps tend to be tender, not painful. As well, many women experience lumpy and tender breasts before their period.

Screening

The Canadian Cancer Society recommends the following guidelines:
- Have a mammogram every two years if you are between the ages of 50 and 69. If you are between the ages of 40 and 49, discuss your risk of breast cancer and the benefits and risks of mammography with your doctor. If you are over 70, talk to your doctor about a screening program for you.
- Have a clinical breast examination by a trained health professional at least every two years if you are over the age of 40.
- Conduct regular breast self-examinations and report any changes to your doctor.

Breast Self-Examination

Many women neglect to do this simple and easy procedure, yet it takes only a few minutes to examine your breasts, and it could save your life. Breast self-examination (BSE) is something that all women should do on a monthly basis three or four days after the end of a menstrual period. At menopause, choose a specific date, such as the first of the month, and perform a BSE on that day each month.

1. Stand in front of a mirror and look at your breasts. Slowly turn from side to side and look for any changes in shape and for rashes or puckers in the skin.
2. Raise your arms over your head and continue looking in the mirror for changes. Put your hands behind your head and look at your breasts and underarm area.
3. Put your palms together, squeeze, and lower your hands to your nose. Again, look for any changes.
4. Feel your breasts with your fingers. Put your fingers together and keep your hand flat (not cupped). Use the pads of your fingers, opposite hand for each breast, and start below the collarbone. Cover the entire breast area using a circular or grid-like pattern, and then do the underarm area. Keep constant contact and pressure.
5. Lie down on your back on a firm surface. Put one hand behind your head and use the opposite hand to check your breast as above.

If you notice any changes in the look or feel of your breasts, see your doctor. Most of the time changes that women find do not indicate cancer, but it is important to have it checked out in order to be sure.

Prevention

According to the Canadian Cancer Society, at least 50 percent of cancers can be prevented through healthy living. Below are some lifestyle choices that can help reduce the risk of breast cancer:

- Eat a diet high in fibre. Flaxseeds, oat bran, fruits, and vegetables are all great sources of fibre. Cruciferous vegetables such as broccoli, cauliflower, kale, and Brussels sprouts contain cancer-fighting nutrients.
- Minimize your intake of saturated fat and avoid trans fats.
- Maintain a healthy body weight.
- Be physically active. Studies show that even moderate physical activity may reduce your risk by 30 to 40 percent. Spend at least 30 minutes on five or more days of the week doing aerobic activities such as brisk walking, cycling, or swimming.
- Limit your alcohol intake to no more than one drink per day, or cut it out altogether.
- Breastfeed your baby. Breastfeeding seems to offer protection against breast cancer, plus it's good for the baby.
- Don't smoke. Smoking and breathing second-hand smoke can increase the risk of breast cancer, along with many other health problems.
- Only use hormone replacement therapy if absolutely necessary and for a short period of time (less than five years).

- Minimize your exposure to chemicals that have been linked to increased cancer risk such as dioxins, phthalates, pesticides, and herbicides. Some of these chemicals are referred to as *xenoestrogens* because they have estrogen-like activity in the body. Dioxins are found most abundantly in farmed fish and in the fumes from incinerated waste. Phthalates are found in plastics, particularly when they are heated or reused, and pesticides and herbicides are concentrated in non-organic produce. For information on chemicals and disease, refer to the CHE Toxicant and Disease Database, http://database.healthandenvironment.org/.

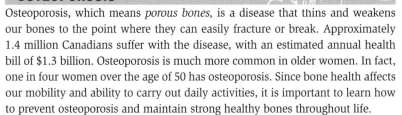

OSTEOPOROSIS

Osteoporosis, which means *porous bones,* is a disease that thins and weakens our bones to the point where they can easily fracture or break. Approximately 1.4 million Canadians suffer with the disease, with an estimated annual health bill of $1.3 billion. Osteoporosis is much more common in older women. In fact, one in four women over the age of 50 has osteoporosis. Since bone health affects our mobility and ability to carry out daily activities, it is important to learn how to prevent osteoporosis and maintain strong healthy bones throughout life.

Bone Basics

Bone is a living tissue; it is in a constant state of growth and deterioration. It consists of a matrix of protein fibers (collagen) hardened with calcium, phosphorus, magnesium, zinc, copper, and other minerals. There is an interconnecting structure that gives bone its strength. On the outside there is a tough, dense rind of cortical bone, and on the inside there is the spongy-looking trabecular bone.

Bone cells called *osteoclasts* are constantly breaking down old bone at the same time that other cells, called *osteoblasts,* are building new bone. The activity of these cells is regulated primarily by the hormones estrogen, testosterone, and parathyroid hormone.

Until we are roughly 30 years old, there is a balance in the activity of osteoclasts and osteoblasts. After that point bone loss usually begins. In women, the rate of loss accelerates for several years after menopause, and then slows again.

The trabecular bone normally looks like a honeycomb, but in those with osteoporosis the spaces in that honeycomb grow larger because more bone is destroyed than replaced. This makes the bones weaker and more susceptible to fractures.

Symptoms of the Silent Thief

Osteoporosis is referred to as the *silent thief* because bone loss can occur slowly over many years and without symptoms until a sudden strain, bump, or fall causes a bone fracture. It most commonly affects bones in the hip, spine, or wrist.

In severe cases, it can cause a collapsed vertebrae leading to symptoms of back pain, loss of height, or spinal deformities.

Bone mineral density (BMD) is a term used to describe the solidity of our bones. This can be determined by a DEXA-scan (dual-energy X-ray absorptiometry). The results are reported as a number that tells us how far off our BMD is from a healthy adult without osteoporosis. For example, a result of –2.5 SD (standard deviation) or greater indicates the presence of osteoporosis. A result between –1 SD to –2.5 SD means there is some bone loss, a condition called osteopenia.

Risk Factors We Can Control

- Diet: Low calcium intake and low vitamin D both contribute to bone loss. High caffeine intake (more than four drinks per day) may also contribute to bone loss.
- Anorexia: Anorexia can cause bone loss.
- Alcohol: High alcohol consumption (more than two drinks per day) increases risk of developing osteoporosis.
- Lack of activity: A sedentary lifestyle increases risk of osteoporosis.
- Smoking: Smoking increases risk of osteoporosis.
- Medications: Prescription medications such as steroids (prednisone) and anticonvulsants can increase risk of osteoporosis.

Risk Factors Beyond Our Control

- Age: Those who are age 65 or older are at increased risk.
- Gender: Women are more susceptible than men.
- Ethnicity: People of Caucasian or Asian descent are at a higher risk of developing osteoporosis.
- Body frame: Those with small, thin bones are more likely to be affected by osteoporosis.
- Family history: Having a parent that suffered with osteoporosis increases risk.
- Previous medical conditions: Medical conditions that affect calcium absorption such as Celiac or Crohn's disease increase risk.
- Osteopenia: Those who have been diagnosed with osteopenia (mild bone loss) are at increased risk.

Medical Management

Proper nutrition and exercise are the cornerstones for osteoporosis prevention, but in some cases drug therapy is necessary to either slow the rate of bone loss or promote bone development. There are a variety of medications that doctors prescribe, such as hormones and bisphosphonates (such as etidronate).

Building Better Bones

Just as we contribute to retirement savings during our working lives to ensure financial stability in later life, we can contribute to our bone stores to prevent osteoporosis. If you already have bone loss, there are still measures you can take to prevent further loss and to strengthen your bones.

Exercise

Weight-bearing activities, which place stress on the bone, help to strengthen bones and improve bone density. Examples include weightlifting, walking, tennis, and dancing. Exercise also increases muscle strength, coordination, and balance. Together, these factors preserve mobility and independence and reduce the risk of injury and fracture. If you have osteoporosis, consult with your doctor before you start exercising and seek guidance from a personal trainer to avoid possible injury.

Nutrition

There are certain vitamins and minerals that are essential to building strong bones, such as calcium, magnesium, and vitamin D. National surveys have found that many people consume less than half of the recommended amount of calcium necessary for healthy bones. For women, the recommended amount is 1000 mg for ages 19 to 50, and 1200 mg for those above 50.

Calcium-rich foods include low-fat dairy (cheese, yogurt, and milk), canned fish with bones (salmon and sardines), dark green vegetables (kale, collards, and broccoli) and calcium-fortified orange juice and soy milk. Three to four servings of dairy products provides about 1200 mg of calcium. One serving equals one cup of milk, ¾ cup yogurt, ½ cup cottage cheese, or a 3 cm cube of hard cheese. Those who fall short of the recommended daily amounts should consider taking a calcium supplement.

Magnesium is required by the enzymes that convert vitamin D into its active form, and also for the proper secretion of hormones that regulate bone health. Women over 30 require 320 mg daily. The best food sources are leafy green vegetables, unrefined grains, nuts, seeds, meat, milk, soybeans, tofu, legumes, and figs.

Vitamin D aids in the absorption of calcium. We produce some vitamin D when our skin is exposed to sunlight. Spending 15 minutes outdoors daily helps your body manufacture the required vitamin D. It is also present in fortified milk products and breakfast cereals, fatty fish, and eggs. For women, the recommended intake is 200 IU for ages 19 to 50, 400 IU for ages 51 to 70, and 600 IU for those above age 70. Individuals with osteoporosis or those who are taking medications that impair vitamin D absorption may require higher amounts.

Soy foods such as tofu, soy milk, roasted soy beans, and soy powders, can also play a role in the prevention of osteoporosis. Soy contains isoflavones, which are plant-based estrogens that protect against bone loss.

Foods to Avoid

Too much caffeine (more than three cups coffee per day) or sodium can increase calcium loss through urination, accelerating bone deterioration. Soft drinks also contribute to bone loss by changing the acid balance in the blood.

Supplements for Bone Health

• Ipriflavone is an isoflavone derivative that is used worldwide for the treatment and prevention of osteoporosis. Numerous studies have found that it prevents bone loss and reduces bone pain caused by osteoporosis and fractures. It is most effective when taken along with calcium.

• Boron, copper, manganese, phosphorus, vitamin K, silicon, and zinc are other nutrients involved in bone formation. In some cases, deficiencies of these substances have been associated with an increased risk of osteoporosis. These nutrients are often included in bone-building supplements along with calcium, magnesium, and vitamin D.

Since individual needs and dosages vary, it is important to consult with a qualified health care practitioner before taking supplements.

Final Thoughts

Osteoporosis is preventable, not inevitable. As you read in this chapter, there are various ways to build strong bones and protect yourself against osteoporosis. A diet that is rich in calcium and vitamin D, regular weight-bearing exercise, and nutritional supplements are key elements in our personal fight against osteoporosis. If we are diligent about maintaining a bone-healthy lifestyle, it is possible to keep the silent thief of osteoporosis at bay.

MENOPAUSE

In a woman's lifetime her body goes through many changes in response to the natural rise and fall of hormones. During the reproductive years, hormones fluctuate in cycles to prepare the body for child bearing. In menopause, ovulation ceases and a woman can no longer conceive naturally. While some women have anxiety about what this phase in life may bring, it is actually a time to be embraced as there is a freedom from monthly hormonal changes and the menstrual period.

The Transition

At birth women have about one million eggs in their ovaries. At puberty ovulation starts; eggs are released by the ovaries each month for the purpose of conception. As the years go by the amount of eggs gradually decline until menopause, when the ovaries shut down and stop producing estrogen and progesterone—the two main female sex hormones. Menopause usually happens naturally as women age, but it can occur for other reasons, such as the removal of both ovaries, or subsequent to radiation or chemotherapy.

Once a woman reaches menopause and the ovaries are in retirement, the adrenal glands, which supply some sex hormones throughout life, become the primary supplier. Women who have poor adrenal function, which can be caused by chronic stress, poor diet, lack of sleep, or excessive caffeine, are not able to provide adequate hormone amounts, and may have more severe menopausal symptoms.

Estrogen can also be produced in the fat cells from androgens. This is why obese women often experience fewer symptoms of estrogen deficiency than thin women.

Am I in Menopause?

The milestone of menopause is reached when a woman goes one year without a menstrual period. The average age for menopause is about 51, but it can occur naturally between ages 40 and 55. The decade or so before menopause is now referred to as peri-menopause. During this time hormone levels fluctuate and the menstrual cycle becomes erratic. Some months you may have a period and others you may not. However, during this time you may still be able to get pregnant.

Symptoms

Some women sail through menopause with no symptoms at all, while others struggle for months or even years. The symptoms can be linked to an imbalance of hormones:

- Low estrogen causes vaginal dryness, incontinence, foggy head, and depression.
- Low progesterone causes low libido, depression, fatigue, foggy head, headache, irritability, memory loss, and fluid retention.
- Low testosterone causes low libido, fatigue, and bone loss.
- Estrogen dominance—a drop in progesterone levels and an accumulation in the body of estrogen-like chemicals called xenoestrogens—causes the same symptoms as those of low progesterone.

Undoubtedly, the most notorious of all menopausal symptoms are hot flashes, which some women refer to as *power surges*. Nearly 75 percent of women experience hot flashes, which vary in duration and intensity. For some women they can be debilitating, as they affect sleep and normal daily activities. The actual cause of hot flashes is unknown. For years it was thought that they were caused by a lack of estrogen. However, we now know that some women with high estrogen levels also get them. In some cultures, such as with Asian women, hot flashes are very rare. Body type is another factor—thin women typically experience more hot flashes because they have fewer fat cells to provide that secondary source of estrogen in menopause. Smoking and drinking alcohol can also increase hot flashes. The good news is that they don't last forever, and there are ways to minimize hot flashes.

Weight gain before or after menopause is another common concern, and there are a variety of factors that may be at play. High estrogen levels, as is common in peri-menopause or among those with estrogen dominance (low progesterone levels), can impair thyroid function. Impaired thyroid function may lead to weight gain because the thyroid gland is involved in regulating your metabolic rate. Weight gain around the waist could be associated with high stress. Stress elevates cortisol levels, which causes fat to accumulate around the mid-section.

You can manage the symptoms of menopause and enjoy good health by addressing the factors that cause hormone imbalance and by following a healthy lifestyle.

Managing Menopause

Years ago hormone replacement therapy was offered to most women in menopause, regardless of whether they had symptoms, as it was thought that hormones could protect against heart disease and osteoporosis. Several large studies conducted over the past 10 years have found that while hormones do help prevent bone loss, they can increase the risk of heart disease, stroke, and breast cancer. For these reasons, hormones are now used only for women experiencing severe symptoms that cannot be helped by other measures, and they are used at low doses for short periods of time (less than five years).

Natural (bio-identical) hormones are becoming more widely used as they are thought to be safer, while still providing the benefits for symptom relief. These products are available in compounding pharmacies, by a doctor's prescription.

Natural Supplements for Menopause

Below is a list of supplements that can offer benefits for the various symptoms and concerns that arise during menopause. It is not recommended that you take all of these products; rather, you should consult with your health care provider to determine which products are most suitable for you and the appropriate dosage.

- Black cohosh is an herb that reduces hot flashes, night sweats, insomnia, nervousness, and irritability.
- Chaste tree berry (Vitex) is an herb that helps balance hormones and is particularly helpful during peri-menopause.
- Fish oils help to protect against heart disease by lowering blood pressure and cholesterol, reducing atherosclerosis, and protecting against heart attack.
- Ginkgo biloba is an herb that helps improve memory and cognitive function by increasing blood flow to the brain. It is also an antioxidant.

- Melatonin is a hormone that regulates our sleep/wake cycles. It is naturally secreted by the body in response to darkness. Supplements of melatonin help to improve sleep quality by reducing the time needed to fall asleep and nighttime waking.
- Multivitamin and mineral complexes are important to ensure all essential nutrients are obtained. Many of the B vitamins play a role in hormone balance, antioxidants help protect against age-related diseases, and minerals are important for heart and muscle function.
- St. John's wort is an herb that helps relieve symptoms of depression, anxiety, and irritability. It is often used along with black cohosh.

Lifestyle Measures

There are a number of lifestyle measures that can greatly improve health during menopause:

- Broccoli, Brussels sprouts, cauliflower, and cabbage contain compounds that help the liver process hormones while reducing the risk of breast cancer. Soy foods (tofu, soy milk, soybeans, soy nuts) contain isoflavones (plant-based estrogens) that help to minimize menopausal symptoms, offer protection against breast cancer, and improve bone health. Flaxseeds are a rich source of fibre, which promotes bowel regularity, reduces the risk of colon and breast cancer, and lowers cholesterol. Flaxseeds also contains lignan (phytoestrogens) that may help reduce menopausal symptoms.
- Stress can make menopausal symptoms more pronounced. Meditation, yoga, and breathing techniques can help reduce stress.
- Regular exercise can improve physical and emotional well-being. Studies have shown that regular exercise reduces the frequency and severity of hot flashes. It also protects against heart disease.
- Smoking can worsen hot flashes and symptoms of anxiety, irritability, and depression.

Final Thoughts

Menopause is a natural experience that should be welcomed as an important milestone in a woman's life. Most of the symptoms of menopause can be managed very effectively with proper lifestyle measures and supplements.

WEIGHT MANAGEMENT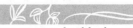

Carrying excess body fat is linked to some of our greatest health threats, namely heart disease, diabetes, and cancer. It can also elevate blood pressure and add stress to the body. Obesity is linked to gall bladder disease, gastro-intestinal disease, sexual dysfunction, osteoarthritis, and stroke. The emotional consequences of obesity can be just as serious: low self-esteem, depression, and anxiety.

It is important to note that if you are overweight or obese, losing even a small amount of weight can improve your health. Studies have shown that losing 10 to 15 percent of excess weight can help reduce blood pressure, blood sugar, and cholesterol. It is important to get your body fat percentage checked. This can be done at a medical centre or health club. The recommended range of body fat for women is 15 to 25 percent.

Apples versus Pears

Research has found that fat on the thighs and hips is less dangerous than fat that accumulates around the mid-section.

Abdominal obesity, or an "apple" shaped body, is associated with more health risks than a "pear" shaped body (larger hips and thighs), because belly fat produces chemicals that trigger inflammation and increase cholesterol and clot formation—all risk factors for heart disease. Belly fat is also associated with insulin resistance, which leads to type 2 diabetes.

To determine whether your mid-section is putting you at risk, check your waist circumference. In women, a measurement of greater than 88 cm (35 inches) represents an increased risk. Being physically active, not smoking, and using unsaturated fat over saturated fat have been shown to *decrease* the risk of developing abdominal obesity.

Factors Affecting Body Weight

In the past it was thought that diet and activity level were the only factors affecting body weight. We now know that this is not the case. Some people can exercise regularly and reduce caloric intake and still not lose weight. And, of course, we all know people who can eat whatever they want and never gain a pound.

Weight gain and obesity are complex conditions, dependent upon various lifestyle, hormonal, biochemical, metabolic, and genetic factors. Some of the most important factors include:

- Basal Metabolic Rate (BMR): The rate at which your body burns calories at rest is called your BMR. Your BMR is dependent on several of the factors listed below, such as activity level and thyroid function.
- Caloric intake: Overeating and consuming more calories than your body uses for energy can result in weight gain—regardless of whether those calories come from fat, carbohydrates, or protein.
- Activity level: Inactivity causes loss of muscle mass, reduced metabolic rate, and increased body fat, whereas regular exercise improves muscle mass and boosts metabolism.

- Stress: Chronic stress can cause weight gain, particularly around the mid-section. Stress increases the production and release of cortisol, a hormone that increases body fat storage. Stress has become a common concern for women today as more women are juggling family, career, and household responsibilities.
- Human growth hormone (HGH): HGH is an important hormone for regulating body weight. Low levels can cause a loss of lean muscle mass and an increase in body fat storage. Levels decline with age, particularly after age 50, causing a shift in our body composition.
- Lack of sleep: Research has found that lack of sleep (less than six hours per night) can raise levels of hormones that increase appetite and decrease levels of HGH.
- Thyroid function: The thyroid gland plays a vital role in controlling metabolism. If your thyroid is low and not functioning optimally, this can reduce your metabolic rate and cause weight gain. Low thyroid is very common in women between the ages of 30 and 50. Symptoms include cold hands and feet, dry skin, hair loss, low libido, constipation, and depression.
- Insulin: When insulin levels are high the body stores more fat and is not able to use fat as a source of energy.
- Genetics: Genetics play a role in determining body type and weight. However, lifestyle factors are more important determinants.
- Sex hormones: High estrogen levels or low testosterone levels are associated with weight gain.
- Serotonin: A chemical messenger in the brain, serotonin regulates satiety (fullness) and appetite. When levels are low we feel hungry, and when they are high we feel satisfied.

Dietary Strategies

Following a healthy diet is very important for those trying to lose weight. Skipping meals or following a fad diet is not the way to go. Instead, follow the nutritional principles for optimum health outlined in Part One of this book. In particular, keep the following principles in mind:

- Eat four to five small meals/snacks daily to keep your metabolism and energy level optimized.
- Watch your portion sizes.
- Avoid processed, refined, and fast foods as they are high in calories and low in nutritional value.
- Ensure adequate protein intake. Protein is essential for building and maintaining lean muscle mass, and the more muscle you have the more calories you burn.

- Fill up on fibre. Fibre is digested slowly so it keeps you feeling more full and also helps balance blood sugar levels.
- Drink eight to 10 glasses of water daily. Water works with fibre to keep you feeling full. It also helps with the removal of toxins and waste.
- Limit alcohol. Alcohol floods the body with empty calories.

Fitness

Regular physical activity is essential to achieving a healthy body weight. Aim for one hour of moderately intense activity daily. If you are currently not active, start slowly and gradually increase your duration and intensity. Follow the guidelines for cardiovascular activities, resistance training, and stretching outlined in Part One of this book.

Other Lifestyle Strategies

- Reduce your stress. Stress can trigger appetite and food cravings and increases the production of cortisol, a hormone that promotes fat storage around the abdomen.
- Aim for seven to nine hours of sleep per night.
- If you find that your eating habits are tied to your emotions, consider counseling or a support group.

Weight-Loss Supplements

There are numerous weight-loss supplements on the market, but only a few have been clinically tested and proven to offer benefits. Here are a few to consider:

- Conjugated linoleic acid (CLA) is a fatty acid that stimulates the breakdown of stored fat, reduces the number of fat cells, and prevents fat storage.
- Fibre helps reduce appetite and cravings, improve blood sugar balance, and promote weight loss.
- Green tea promotes weight loss by increasing the rate of calorie burning. It may also help reduce appetite and food cravings.
- Hydroxycitric Acid (HCA) is a compound derived from the fruit *Garcinia cambogia*, which supports weight loss by reducing appetite, enhancing the breakdown of fat, and reducing fat storage.
- Phase 2 is a white kidney bean extract that reduces the breakdown of starch into sugar, lowers after-meal sugar levels, and promotes fat loss.

Weighing In

If you have decided to lose weight, set reasonable goals and make small, gradual changes to your lifestyle. Be consistent with your exercise program, eat healthily, and make sure you get adequate sleep. Most importantly, be patient. It takes time to lose weight, but the rewards are worthwhile.

Part Three

FINANCIAL HEALTH

Planning for the future not only requires making healthy decisions for your body and soul, it requires a sound financial plan to help you reach your goals. This chapter talks about the process involved in financial planning, and where to get professional planning advice.

Financial Planning

Developing a financial plan can be daunting if you have never completed one. Most people welcome help with their savings and investments, life and health insurance, and disability protection. The good news is there are trained professionals who can help you build a plan that will help you achieve your dreams.

Where Do I Begin?

Getting started is more important than getting it right the first time. The following steps will help guide you in building your plan. A financial advisor can help you develop a plan if you need assistance, or they can review a plan you have created to ensure you haven't missed an important step.

1. **Assess where you are now.**
   Begin by making a list of all your major assets, your expenses, and your income.
2. **Set future goals.**
   Next, set specific achievable goals. Be sure to allow yourself time to really think about what you want to achieve, when you want to retire, and what lifestyle you want to maintain throughout your life. Remember to estimate how much money you think you will need to save, how you will protect your assets, and how much time you have to achieve your financial goals.
3. **Manage financial risk.**
   This is an important step many people fail to recognize as essential to their financial plan. Have you ever thought about the impact a disability, a critical illness, or the death of your spouse would have on your financial future? It is important you have the proper protection in place to ensure your plan can succeed should the unexpected happen. When you prepare for the worst, you get more pleasure from the best life offers, knowing that everyone is protected. Including insurance protection in your financial plan helps to prepare for the unknown that could affect your financial wealth and security. Make sure you also have a will and have appointed a power of attorney. Planning allows you to take charge of the risks in your control and protects you against those that are not.

A will gives you the opportunity to put the right person in charge as executor and to designate who will inherit your assets and who will care for your children. With a power of attorney, you allow someone you trust to manage your property and your personal care if you become unable to act due to illness or disability.

4. **Seek good advice.**
Once you have created your plan, have a professional review it. You may want to consult your accountant, lawyer, and financial advisor to ensure there are no gaps in your plan and to provide you with the calculations you need to ensure your plan will really help you achieve your goals.
5. **Implement your plan.**
Once you have set your goals, take action. Implement your financial plan to achieve the goals you have set. Put your plan into action and see your hard work deliver as you expected.
6. **Take stock.**
Most importantly, take time at least once a year to review your financial plan, to seek advice for answers to questions you may have, and to determine if you are on track to achieving your goals. Creating a financial plan is only the beginning. You must keep your plan in-line with your life. Some of the life changes that impact your plan include the following:
   • You get married or divorced.
   • You have a baby or your child becomes ill.
   • You purchase a new home or pay off a mortgage.
   • You change jobs, location, or country.

Financial planning is an ongoing task. As your life evolves, so should your plans. Be sure to carefully monitor your plan as you reach new milestones in your life.

Good Advice Is Essential to a Good Financial Plan
A good financial advisor will take the time to learn about your personal situation and to provide the services and follow-through you need to integrate your financial plan. Most importantly, a good financial advisor knows how to listen, will not judge your decisions, and will offer suggestions on how you can reach your goals in your own way.

Proper Planning Ensures Optimum Financial Health
A solid financial plan is as important for your future as making healthy choices. A plan can lessen the financial risks of living a long life and help you value

the present. By following a few simple steps, you can create a plan that will help you achieve your goals and protect your dreams. Don't forget to speak to a professional about your financial plan to ensure you have covered all of the bases. Most importantly, enjoy the process of taking charge of your financial well-being today and in the future.

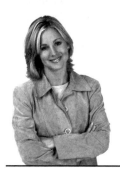

ABOUT THE AUTHOR

Sherry Torkos, BSc, Phm

Sherry Torkos is a pharmacist, author, and certified fitness instructor. She received her Bachelor of Science degree in Pharmacy from the Philadelphia College of Pharmacy and Science in 1992 and practices in the Niagara region of Ontario.

As a leading health expert, she has delivered hundreds of lectures to medical professionals and the public. She is frequently interviewed on radio and TV talk shows throughout North America and abroad.

She has authored eight books, including *Winning at Weight Loss* (Wiley, 2005), *The Benefits of Berries* (Bearing, 2005), *Proven Natural Solutions for Depression* (Wiley, 2004), and *Breaking the Age Barrier* (Penguin Books, 2003).

For more information visit www.sherrytorkos.com